The Ultimate Guide To Doubling & Tripling Your Dental Practice Production

...

How To Build An Unstoppable Dental Practice With The Freedom To Enjoy It!

Wendy Briggs, RDH & John Meis, DDS, FAGD, DICOI

Publisher: The Team Training Institute, www.TheTeamTrainingInstitute.com

ISBN-13: 978-1507858363
ISBN-10: 1507858361

The Most Incredible Free Gift Ever….

Claim Your $2,998 Dental Practice Growth Gift

Valid for 1 60-minute Practice Analysis Amplifier. The Team Training Institute will analyze your current practice and provide you with a roadmap to implement all 5 key areas of growth in your practice.

To CLAIM Your Gift:
www.HowToDoubleProduction.com/freegift

TABLE OF CONTENTS

Part 2: Systematize For Success

Part 3: Grow With Profits

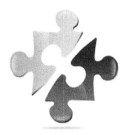

Preface

What If Everything You Have Been Told About Building A Dental Practice Was Wrong?

You have finally found it…

The one place (The Team Training Institute) designed for the dentist who wants to grow their practice by following the footsteps of those that have done it, who are in the trenches, who know exactly what you are going through.

This is a road map of sorts.

See all Dentists at all levels are stuck – you are either growing or dying – there is no middle. Which leaves us with a GREAT OPPORTUNITY. There is so much yet to learn.

From the brand new dentist who just graduated dental school to the guy/gal who has been practicing for the last 50 years – we are all looking at getting better at what we do – always looking for that little edge. It's what makes us successful.

We are here to help you…to provide you with the resources to master not only providing a world-class experience for your patients   BUT to create YOUR Ideal practice. The practice that provides you and your family with the lifestyle of your dreams, and the freedom to enjoy it.

My name is Wendy Briggs, and I have been a registered dental hygienist for over 25 years. When I first started out, I was happy with a status quo. I saw patients, did my job and never really questioned the system. I was making good money for the practice – but nowhere even close the potential of where it could be!

But something else bothered me even more. I had an arsenal of wonderful treatments to help my patients have a healthy mouth, *but I was hardly using any of it.*

The dentist I worked for was busy drilling and filling. Every day it was the same basic routine…. and as a team we were using just a fraction of the latest tools. I knew there had to be a better way.

So I took action and made a **list of everything I knew to be true about the practice**:

✓ The dentist had excellent skills

✓ We, the hygienists, were the frontline of the practice

✓ We weren't using ¾ of the tools at our disposal

✓ The dentist sort of haphazardly tried to offer more procedures (he wasn't very comfortable with "selling") *with little results*

✓ Our hygiene department procedures and scripting weren't consistent with *every* patient

My interest in improving oral health became an obsession. Every day I would brainstorm for a better way, by thinking like a business owner… and improving patient care and bottom-line profits were the only measurement tools I used to rate every idea.

And one day…I had one of those Ah-hah discovery moments!

Since hygienists are on the front line of almost every dental practice…and since hygienists spend the most time with patients…and since hygienists have the most tools available to help patients have healthier, more attractive smiles…*then here's the million dollar question…*

Why weren't we maximizing our strengths to produce amazing profits for the practice?!?

I spent the next however many years working to perfect a system that would turn the hygiene department into a profitable MACHINE.

Where you could plug in a new patient and be <u>guaranteed</u> that they would receive the highest of care AND your practice would optimize the production of every chair.

First, I tested my ideas on my own, at the practice where I worked.

Then, through my inner-circle (my network of friends who are working hygienists in practices across the U.S.) we started beta-testing my exact same scripting at the practices where they worked.

<u>**Bottom line: by approaching hygiene like a business owner**</u>, and by consistently asking the same, scripted questions… within the first 30 days…

Hygiene production doubled, tripled even quadrupled in every instance

The doctor I worked for was stunned and amazed at the financial turn around. He encouraged me to keep going.

So that's exactly what I did. In fact, over the next 3 years, I perfected a <u>ridiculously easy to implement system</u> that (I will walk you through the entire system in Chapters 3, 4, &5)

> ➤ **Skyrockets the bottom-line** net profit by an average of $27,432 in the first 60 days of the practice because this is newly uncovered, sheer profit!

> ➤ **Empowers the hygienist** to guide the course of the patient's treatment and create new opportunities for same-day, in-office treatments and at-home treatments! Translation: more revenue, more perio diagnosed, more referrals. *AND*...I could increase my daily hygiene production right on the spot with ease!

> ➤ **Creates the happiest of patients** because they become a part of keeping their teeth and gums healthy which means less time in the chair and less pain for them and they also get the beautiful smiles that they've always dreamed about!

> ➤ **Allows the hygienist to spend quality time** with the patients to increase production and not rush more patients through the operatory!

This system became a **WIN-WIN-WIN** for everyone.

I have since taught this system to over 3,718 offices in 12 countries around the world, and I continue to teach it – In short it works.

But I still wasn't satisfied…. I knew that this was just the first step in creating the dental practice that every dentist dreams of.

Dr. John Meis

Then I went into the office of Dr. John Meis in Sioux City Iowa, and it was like finding my dentist clone. Dr. John had cracked the code for optimizing the dentist's production and creating a practice that is bulletproof, (or TIGER-proof) just like I had cracked the code in hygiene production.

Let me tell you a little about Dr. John, he was destined to be a dentist… his father was a dentist, his fathers' father was a dentist, and his fathers' fathers' father was a dentist (that makes him a 4th generation dentist, if you lost count.) … So he figured that being a dentist sounded like a pretty good job.

But his practice was not always what I saw – he struggled and suffered through frustration and the misery of an under-performing practice that was constantly struggling just to get a head.

He had bought into just about every consultant, every gimmick for getting new patients, for getting referrals, for training his team. He had spent hundreds of thousands of dollars on seminars, and marketing products, and coaching.

Then one night he woke up with chest pains – as a 28-year-old guy who was in great shape   that is not what you expected when you go to sleep.

He realized that every day he was feeling more and more fatigued, things that were once easy were becoming very difficult, and things just kept getting worse.

His doctor sent him to another doctor, who sent him to another doctor, who sent him to another doctor, and he eventually ended up at the University of Iowa Hospital, talking to a transplant specialist. Talk about SCARY.

They finally diagnosed him with cardiomyopathy, and as quickly as it came on it disappeared and he has been symptom free for over 25 years... BUT it was during this scare that he realized he was not in a financial position not to work.

What would happen to his wife? What would happen to his 2 young children? What would happen to his dental practice? What would happen to his team? Questions and feelings that I bet, many of you reading this wonder every day.

Because of this scare, he decided to get serious. He decided he was going to crack the code and figure out how he could use his practice to not only make a good living, but to become financially secure as quickly as possible, and leave a legacy for his children.

For the next 8 years he went out and got as much continuing education as physically possible. He became a Fellow of the Academy of General Dentistry and a Diplomat of the International Congress of Implantologists, the president of his local dental society, and the president of the state AGD…. And where did it get him?

Nowhere…. Nothing…. Collections = down, profitability = down. He was a smarter, better dentist … but his practice wasn't showing it.

His Eureka Moment

"I was operating under the wrong structure, and I wasn't thinking about my practice as a business!"

So, he started to study:

- Practices that were doing over 50 Million a year

- The really high producers (over $200K/month personal production)

- Those that had Million dollar net incomes

You would think that they were all 3 the same people –

but they weren't! They were 3 separate groups.

Dr. John determined that there were 11 productive practice principles that applied to those 3 groups and he set out to build his practice using these 11 principles.

You can download a copy of the 11 practice principles at: www.TheTeamTrainingInstitute.com/11principles

Within 3 years, he was producing over $225K/month in personal production, and his flagship practice was in the top 1% of all dental practices.

It was at this time, that I met Dr. John. In fact, he was a little skeptical that I could double his hygiene, since they were already hyper producers. The month following my visit and the implementation of my hygiene system, his <u>hygiene was up 73%.</u>

We spent one lunch going over the principles that we both used to grow and I realized that he was the missing piece in my puzzle and he realized that I was the missing piece to his.

Together we created the Team Training Institute and made it our mission to show dentists how they too, can double their production, establish their practice and have the freedom to enjoy it!

How do we do this?

It's a 5-Step SYSTEM that any doctor can follow, and the best part about it? We will show you how you can create the income needed to grow your practice from what you already have.

This means there is no output of money, until you have made the revenue and determined to re-invest that money in your practice. That's the beauty of this system ☺

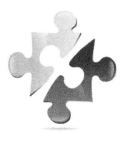

Part 1

Optimize
Production

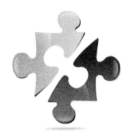

CHAPTER 1

Why You Don't Have A New Patient Problem

This is a warning: There is little profit or success in just learning a new tactic to drive new patients or implementing a script for case acceptance in and of itself.

There is enormous profit, reduced stress, and a better patient experience in understanding HOW these tactics apply to your ideal practice.

This might shock you but you **DO NOT have a new patient problem**.

There is NEVER going to be a shortage of new patients, let me start by explaining that you don't have a "new patient problem" – the problem is that most practices don't know how to optimize the patients that they have…

80% of the revenue that you will get from a patient comes in the first 18 months they are in your practice – do you have a bullet proof system to ensure that you are the dentist that is receiving the revenue?

There is little benefit in bringing in hordes of new patients if they are simply falling out the back door.

The 5-Step System That Has Taken More Dentists to the Top 1% Than Ever Before

There are only 5 steps that you need to put your income into the top 1% of all Dentists and ensure that you and your family no longer have to worry about money, your staff no longer needs to worry about the practice, and your patients will always know that you are providing high-quality dental care for their long-term health. They are:

1. Optimize Production
2. Create Systems
3. Build a Management Team
4. Tiger Proof
5. Replace Your Salary with Profits

These are the 5-steps that we have used to take practices from the brink of bankruptcy to over $1M in revenue; to take a $1M practice to $5M and every practice in between.

We have also helped doctors build additional locations and be profitable in an average of 7 months. And we will reveal everything to you here today.

Let's get started....

CHAPTER 2

How To Double Production Starting Tomorrow

Step #1: Optimize Production

We all have opportunity to add immediate revenue and profit to our current practice. Without adding any additional marketing costs, without having to add any new patients. Simply by utilizing our current schedule and providing our patients with what they need, and what they ask for.

But this isn't just about adding in a new script or offering services … if you are not focused on creating an optimal environment this won't be successful. In fact this is likely why this has failed in the past.

Early I brought up the controversial statement that you

don't have a "new patient problem." You might have a business model problem, you might have a capacity problem, you might have case acceptance problem, and you might have staff problems….

But you **DO NOT** have a new patient problem.

Before I explain – take a moment to rate your practice:

If I called your office today as a new patient, are you able to see me today?	Y	N
If I was diagnosed with perio today – can you see me within 7 days?	Y	N
If I am presented with a treatment plan for a filling or crown – how soon could you see me?	Today	Not Today
Do you currently have an 80% acceptance rate for adult fluoride?	Y	N
Do you currently place sealants on all open grooves regardless of age and insurance?	Y	N

Are you currently offering de-sensitizing treatments when patients complain of sensitivity or if they jump, flinch or show obvious discomfort during their cleaning?	Y	N
Is your hygiene production currently above $200/hour?	Y	N

If you have more answers in the right hand column vs. the left-hand column, I have good news and bad news for you.

The Good News: You can quickly and easily optimize your production and drive an in flux of cash and revenue into your practice. And the best part…everything that you need to do that, is inside of your practice RIGHT NOW.

The Bad News: Every day that you are not optimizing your production, you are losing a massive amount of cash and revenue from your practice.

I break "Optimizing Production" down into 2 categories; Optimize Hygiene Production and Optimize Clinical Production.

Let's start with Optimizing Hygiene Production….

I have defined 3 roles that a hygienist must utilize to maximize their production.

I start here, because the Hygienist is really the backbone of the dental practice. If we build our practice around this premise and we maximize these 3 roles, you will see that everything else will fall into place.

3 Key Roles of the Hygiene Provider

Preventive Therapist: As the "preventive therapist" the hygienist becomes the source of information regarding the menu of preventive services. When we use the full menu of preventative services (regardless of age and insurance) we are in fact providing a much higher level of patient care, and a level of care that our patients want and need.

Periodontal Therapist: Its not just about saving teeth anymore, it's now about saving lives. Patients are at much greater risk of other serious medical disorders if we do not address their periodontal health – and this starts while in the hygiene chair.

Patient Treatment Advocate: I mentioned earlier that the backbone of the dental practice is the Hygienist. This is why; I define 'Patient Treatment Advocate' as a key role. This key role is responsible for moving restorative dentistry onto the doctor's side. When we maximize this role, we see case acceptance skyrocket.

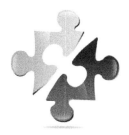

CHAPTER 3

How To Maximize The Preventative Therapist Role

People like to be involved in decisions regarding their health, and their dental health is no different. Gone are the days of 'lecturing' and 'scolding.' Patients have choices and they are not afraid to go elsewhere.

Our job as a Hygiene provider should be to advocate for the dental health of our patients. In doing so, we also provide the dental practice with maximum potential for revenue.

Our goal is to serve all patients at the highest level and the high production naturally follows. But as a business owner, **I know that what is measured and managed will improve**. So, here are 3 key metrics that I look at for this role:

1. **Adult Fluoride Acceptance Rate**: Most practices have a fluoride acceptance rate under 10%. You should have a minimum of 80%, most of the practices that we work with see 90%-95% acceptance of adult fluoride treatments.

2. **Sealant Acceptance Rate**: Regardless of age or insurance, if the tooth indicates that a sealant is the optimal treatment, that should be presented to the patient. How often are we placing sealants? My goal is 4 sealants/day

3. **De-sensitizing agent acceptance rate**: If more than 85% of all adults complain of sensitive teeth, we should be taking the opportunity to provide a bonded agent that will both seal and protect the vulnerable Class V area where recession has occurred.

What is the best way to maximize the acceptance of these procedures? The best thing that we can do is to engage our patients and walk with them through their journey.

The more that we can involve them in this journey and have them making the decisions the higher of an acceptance rate we will have when presenting our solutions.

It all starts with how we set up the visit. At every opportunity possible, we want to engage our patients and have them coming to the conclusion in their head that they are best served with a procedure or service.

What do I mean by this? Take for example probing. It's a vital part of our exam, but have you maximized the potential of this?

I start all of my tissue health assessments, or periodontal probing with a conversation designed to help the patient know what I am looking for.

"I am going to check your tissues for infection. This helps us detect any problems or disease in your gums. You will hear me saying a series of numbers for each tooth, and Chelsea here is going to record the findings for us. A 1-3 means that the tissue is healthy, a 4 means infection is present, and 5 indicates that the infection has already spread to the bone."

Why would I do this?

Because now the patient is hearing my exam, and when they hear 4 and 5's they immediately ask, *"What do we need to do to fix that?"*

And now, when I present that we will need to do some kind of periodontal therapy they have the data to back that up, and were already in the mind-set that they needed to do something different.

They are coming to us looking for a solution, where as before (without this knowledge) they felt that we were just trying to 'sell' them something they didn't need.

I have a script and a system for each and every procedure, and all of my scripts are created to maximize patient acceptance.

Let's take a look at Fluoride:

92% of Dentists are getting less than 74% acceptance with adult fluoride

Most often fluoride is presented something like this (if at all),

> *"We should probably talk about a fluoride treatment, but it isn't covered by your insurance."*

And then we wonder why they don't accept.

When we simply change our language and use these 3 specific steps for presenting fluoride we drive the acceptance rate through the roof:

Step #1: New research has shown _____

The first part is really important, especially for hygienists that aren't currently offering fluoride consistently to adults.

Many practices routinely use fluoride with children because that is when insurance will pay for it. Too often, we don't give our adult patients compelling enough reasons to do fluoride, and we may not even offer it at all.

If you are trying to offer fluoride to adults now and you

haven't in the past, I have found the best way is to start by saying *"new research shows"*.

This is critical for those practices that have not offered fluoride as a part of the preventive care appointment.

"New Research shows that for patients who consistently have a professionally applied fluoride treatment, we can see up to 75% fewer new cavities. This is huge for patients who are always struggling with decay."

Step #2: Here is why fluoride would be good for you today _____

The second step is to share with the patient specific reasons that you feel fluoride would benefit them.

The more specific you can be about what you see in their mouth the better! If they have exposed root surfaces, and dry mouth, they are at a very high risk for decay.

We know how vulnerable those areas are, we need to bring that to their attention.

If they have crown margins, large fillings or many restorations, talk about how fluoride can help protect their investment.

They have spent money and time in rebuilding their mouth and fluoride will help prevent recurrent decay and failure of their dental work.

Step #3: Bad news, insurance won't help with the cost – Good news, it's only $XX

The third step is to let the patient know that there is both good news and bad news about fluoride.

Their dental insurance company will not help with the cost.

That is the bad news.

The good news is that topical application of fluoride is very affordable. It is not an expensive procedure.

Especially when compared with crowns and other restorations.

Many patients see that investing in fluoride even if it's an out-of-pocket expense makes good financial sense.

We need to help them see the value in investing in topically applied fluoride.

So, again here are the steps for increasing fluoride acceptance:

Step #1: New research has shown _____

Step #2: Here is why fluoride would be good for you today _____

Step #3: Bad news, insurance won't help with the cost –

Good news, it's only $xx

Doesn't it sounds better when you say…

"Susan, are you aware that new research has shown that if we do a fluoride varnish every time we polish your teeth, that we can reduce future cavities? We can minimize future decay by as much as 75%. Earlier you mentioned that you were frustrated with always having problems with your teeth. Let's turn that around. Fluoride varnish can help us do that."

"**Everyone has a 95% chance of experiencing caries in the pits and fissures of their teeth, if sealants aren't used**" - The ADA

Because of this, it is a service that many people would like – but are unaware is even available.

We know that early stage cavities and incipient decay are stopped by sealants. But many have been hesitant because the beginning materials were not nearly as good and our procedures were not nearly as good as they are today.

We now have, caries detection technology. We have the Diagnodent, the Spectra, Soprocare Cameras and even the CariVu. As technology continues to improve, we will have even better tools to aid us in detection of decay.

A few years ago, we wouldn't have thought of doing a

sealant on a adult, but with the challenges that we are seeing in patients; medications that cause xerostomia, and other risk factors and with the enhancement of the technology we are able to make a more educated determination of which teeth would be good candidates for sealants.

Our standard of care is now to recommend sealants on all posterior teeth, NOT just those that insurance will pay for. Insurance companies only pay for sealants on children, but that doesn't mean that sealants don't benefit adults.

Dr. David Gore a Prosthodontist and the director of the restorative dentistry department at the University of Kentucky said that for adults age 40 and over sealants maybe the treatment of choice because of rapidly changing medical conditions.

There was also a longevity study completed by Simonsen that said a one-time placement of a sealant could provide a benefit for 15 years.

After 15 years there is a 54% reduction in decay. If you place a sealant and monitor it and maintain it, it can reduce decay by 74% over that 15-year period.

This new research has many dentists re-thinking about how they are utilizing sealants. When good protocol is used, combined with the latest technology, sealants can be a valuable procedure for all ages.

I often challenge hygienists to find at least four sealants

a day in their practice. If a hygienist were to place four sealants on average every day, this adds up to a hefty amount of increased productivity. Not to mention the number of teeth we are protecting each day!

This is why I love to help grow practices. I find ways that they can serve their patients at a higher level while increasing productivity and profitability.

Everyone wins.

When we change our sealant approach, we also stress the value of doing same-day sealants. Patients of today are looking for convenience, and the more often we can provide that for them the more successful we will be.

Over 80% of the adult population suffers from sensitive teeth

Hypersensitivity affects 45 million adults in the US alone.

However in many dental practices we don't consistently offer a bonded solution for someone with sensitive teeth.

This is most likely because many of the products we have used in the past didn't last long term.

Many of our desensitizing agents were designed to go underneath a restoration. When acting as a stand-alone de-sensitizer, they didn't last long enough for us to justify the fee.

Now we have several exciting options that we can use that are proven to provide a benefit for up to three years.

Our extremely sensitive patients really appreciate us solving this problem for them.

The bonded service also protects that vulnerable area from decay, giving the patient the double benefit of no more pain, and protection.

When de-sensitizing agents are presented in the right frame, we have an 89.9% acceptance rate.

The script that I use for this, with an 89.9% acceptance is as follows:

"We have an exciting new service that can help immediately remove the pain and discomfort from your sensitive tooth. It also protects it over time. It's actually easier if I show you how it works rather than try to explain to you how it works. Let's do this, we can try it on your most sensitive tooth. If it doesn't work, you don't pay. If it does work, it's only $29."

I have yet to write-off a treatment. Now, the key … once I have applied the treatment I then say,

"If you start to notice sensitivity creeping back, most likely you have had more recession in the area."

I have opened the loop and started the conversation in their mind, that if they start to feel sensitivity again, they are likely experiencing additional dental problems. This is key for future treatment and future treatment acceptance.

It's not what you say …
it's how you say it.

Framing your conversations so that the benefit to the patients are crystal clear and ensuring that everyone in your office, this includes the Hygienists, the financial coordinator, the front desk team and even you the doctor, are in agreement and following the same script when offering any service, is the key to your success.

So what can maximizing this role do for your practice? Let's take a look at some conservative numbers; let's say you add;

➤ 8 Fluoride treatments a day at $25 = $3,200 a month and $38,400 a year

➤ 4 sealants a day at $45 = $2,880 a month and $34,600 a year

➤ 4 desensitizing agents a day @$39 = $2,496 a month and $29,952 a year

Combined that is a potential $102,952 PER HYGIENIST increase in just hygiene production – and just utilizing the 3 key metrics in the preventative therapist role.

One of the best tools, I use to build value for

preventive services is CAMBRA. Caries Management by Risk Assessment.

The ADA has been recommending that we treat all patients utilizing this for some time now, but most practices don't.

It really is challenging to find the time to do everything there is to do.

Many practices don't have a system in place for doing risk assessment. We know how important this is, but the ADA's survey is three pages long!

Dentists and hygienists alike get excited when I share the tool I use to facilitate the risk assessment conversation in dental practices in just 90 seconds. (and I'll share it with you in just a few pages)

How at risk are your patients?

You might be surprised! It is often stunning when we look at the amount of sugar and the PH levels in the drinks that are common amongst patients.

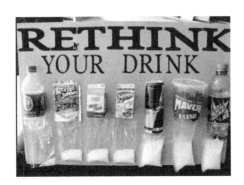

Product	ACID PH LOW=Bad	SUGAR per 12 oz
Pure Water	7.00 Neutral	0
Dasani Water/ Aquafina Water	3.0 5.0	0
Diet Coke	3.39	
Red Wine	3.3	0
Mountain Dew	3.22	11.0 tsp
Gatorade	2.95	3.3 tsp
Pepsi	2.49	9.8 tsp
Coke	2.63	9.3 tsp

Even those that are choosing water, will be surprised at the PH levels of today's bottled water

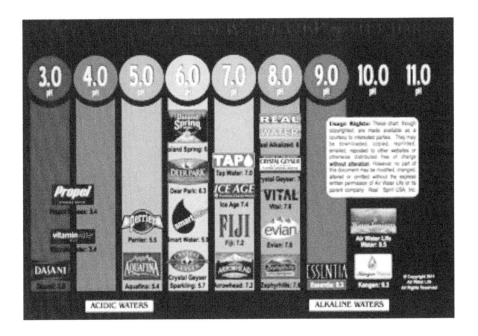

What constitutes "high risk" for adult patients?

The ADA defines "high risk" as:

- 3 or more lesions in the last 3 years
- Suboptimal fluoride exposure
- Xerostomia or Dry Mouth
- Have multiple factors that may increase caries risk

In addition, we have to be aware of the additional items that may increase patients' caries risk. Things like….

- High titers of cariogenic bacteria
- Prolonged nursing (bottle or breast)
- Development of or acquired enamel defects
- Multi-surface restorations
- Chemo/radiation therapy
- Eating disorders
- Cariogenic diet
- Active orthodontic treatment
- Restoration overhangs and open margins
- Plus many more

When we have a risk assessment conversation with patients and use the brochure below, it's like putting prevention on steroids. Most patients don't SEE a need for the preventative services, and it's our job to SHOW them the need and this does exactly that.

In using a tool like this, the conversation can take place in 90 seconds or less! Without using a tool like this, it takes 3x as a long if it happens at all.

PROACTIVE SOLUTIONS

HIGH RISK:

If you are at high risk for dental decay, here are some steps we recommend that can help to minimize your risk.

- Preventive Cavity Screening X-rays every 6 months. (Many insurance companies provide a benefit for this)
- Topical Fluoride Treatment every time you have your teeth polished (reduces cavities by as much as 75%)
- Preventive Sealants on all exposed grooves, regardless of age (ADA states 95% chance of cavities in grooves where sealants are NOT used)
- Minimize sugar intake, especially between meals
- Avoid sugary or Low PH beverages
- Use prescription strength toothpaste and mouth rinses at home to help reduce bacteria content
- Use a Power Toothbrush, and floss as recommended
- Professional Checkup and Cleaning as recommended

MODERATE RISK:

- Preventive Cavity Screening X-rays every 6-12 months. (Many insurance companies provide a benefit for this)
- Topical Fluoride Treatment every time you have your teeth polished (reduces cavities by as much as 75%)
- Preventive Sealants on all exposed grooves, regardless of age (ADA states 95% chance of cavities in grooves where sealants are NOT used)
- Minimize sugar intake, especially between meals
- Avoid sugary or Low PH beverages
- Use prescription strength toothpaste and mouth rinses at home to help reduce bacteria content if recommended
- Use a Power Toothbrush, and floss as recommended
- Professional Checkup and Cleaning as recommended

LOW RISK:

- Preventive Cavity Screening X-rays as recommended.
- Topical Fluoride Treatment as recommended.
- Home care as recommended
- Professional Checkup and Cleaning as recommended

WHAT YOU SHOULD KNOW ABOUT DENTAL X-RAYS

Recently there have been several stories in the media about Dental X-rays. If one didn't know any better, they might take away the message that dental x-rays are bad.

The reality is, that our technology has already solved the issue of high radiation in x-rays. The radiation exposure in cavity detecting x-rays is remarkably low.

To give you some perspective, the American Nuclear Society says that the average radiation level per person per year is 620 millirems (mrems) per year. Safe allowable dose for nuclear plant workers, or those exposed to radiation in their work is 5,000 mrems per year. Here are some examples of other common exposures to radiation:

- 2 hours in a jet plane = 1 mrem
- Living in a stone or adobe house = 7 mrem per year
- 1 pack of cigarettes each day = 36 mrem per year
- Whole body CT scan = 1000 mrem
- 1 bitewing or PA dental x-ray = .08 mrem

This may help you understand why we still feel the benefits our patients receive from x-rays far outweigh the minimal exposure of radiation. Preventive cavity detection x-rays are extremely beneficial in early detection and treatment of cavities.

© 2012 Hygiene Diamonds

PROACTIVE PREVENTION PROGRAM

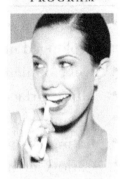

BEAUTIFUL, HEALTHY SMILES, FOR LIFE!

"A patient's risk for developing caries is a moving target."
-The American Dental Association

Many of our patients express concern over having cavities. In fact, Dental caries remains the most common threat to early childhood oral health. It is not just children who are at risk for cavities, however. Many adults also face higher risk due to medical health issues, dietary habits and side effects from common medications.

"Considerable benefit could be achieved if people at high risk levels could be identified before cavities develop." National Institute of Health

The good news is, with appropriate preventive care, we can help to reduce your risk of cavities. The following questions will help us determine what your personal risk status is for decay. With this information, we will both be more effective in preventing future problems.

We take our role in your dental health seriously, and hope to be able to care for your smile for many years to come.

CARIES RISK ASSESSMENT:

HIGH

MODERATE

LOW

CARIES RISK ASSESSMENT SURVEY

Patient Name: _____ Age: ____ Date: ____

Please circle the answers that apply

Low Risk = only conditions in "Low Risk" column present; Moderate Risk = only conditions in "Low" and/or "Moderate Risk" columns present; High Risk = one or more conditions in the "High Risk" column present.

DENTAL CONDITIONS	HIGH	MODERATE	LOW
Plaque/Calculus	Generalized	Localized	Minimal
Visible Cavitations	Yes		No
Cavity in the last 3 Years	Yes		No
Dry Mouth	Yes		No
Exposed Roots	Yes		No
Deep Pits or Fissures	Yes		No
Radiographic Cavities	Yes		No
White Spot Lesions	Yes		No
Appliances Present	Yes		No

MEDICAL HISTORY	HIGH	MODERATE	LOW
GERD	Yes		No
Sjogren's Syndrome	Yes		No
Hyposalivary Meds	Yes		No
Radiation Therapy	Yes		No

HABITS	HIGH	MODERATE	LOW
Snacks between meals	3 + times	1-3 times	Infrequent
Soda or low PH beverage	Yes	Infrequent	No
Recreational Drugs	Yes		No

PROTECTIVE	HIGH	MODERATE	LOW
Flouridated water	No		Yes
Flouridated toothpaste	No		Yes
Fluoride mouthrinse		No	Yes
Xylitol gum/mints		No	Yes
Other protective rinses		No	Yes

AND now, if we have CAMBRA documentation, we are able to submit and possibly even receive payment from insurance companies at a greater level.

To download a FREE copy of this brochure and access my FREE training on how this one tool accounts for 90% of my case acceptance and how I can do it all in 90 seconds of less go to:
www.TheTeamTrainingInstitute.com/risk-assessment-brochure

CHAPTER 4

How To Maximize the Periodontal Therapist Role

The second role of the hygienist is that of a Periodontal Therapist.

Many consultants and hygiene educators focus heavily on periodontal therapy, as it is a critical component in the life of a dental hygienist.

However, it is not uncommon to see a practice that is still treating periodontal infection today with the same strategies and technology that they were using 5 years ago. Sometimes even 10 years ago.

This is truly alarming! Many things have changed. We have better tools, better science about what causes periodontal infection, and how to drastically reduce it. We know so much more about the Oral-Systemic link, and serious health risks that exist with the presence of inflammation in the body.

We have laser techniques, Oral DNA testing methods, better homecare products, and additional resources like Arestin and other adjunctive options for patients.

If we are truly maximizing potential in our role as a Periodontal Therapist, we are seeing periodontal disease, talking about it and treating it.

We should have extremely high acceptance rates for these advanced services, <u>supervised neglect is not an option</u>.

We discuss Periodontal Disease with existing patients, as well as New Patients, and we are treating it with every available weapon in our arsenal.

I review hundreds of Practice Analysis reports every year as a recommended consulting partner for Henry Schein Dental. I am asked to evaluate how periodontal services are being performed and it is stunning to see how often our perception of how perio is being treated is so different from the reality!

When most dentists are asked what percentage of their patients should be receiving periodontal care. They will respond, 25% or even 40%.

When we look at actual utilization of these codes, the reality is that only 1.9% of their patients received periodontal care in the last year.

My take on this is … I don't believe that we are not recognizing and discussing the care that patients need. I believe that the patients don't understand the need and therefore are not moving forward with treatment.

I use a simple approach to gaining a higher level of acceptance for Periodontal Services. I talk about utilizing technology to provide a measure of proof.

Use your intra-oral cameras, especially the incredible Perio Mode feature available on the Soprocare camera. (My new favorite!) to help the patient see for themselves what is happening in their mouth.

I then follow up with 3 simple things we need to do to treat the infection in their mouth.

"To clear up this infection we need to do these 3 things…."

I then go on to explain the three steps needed to clear up the infection:

#1: *"We need to do a deep, more aggressive cleaning than you've had in the past."* **And then I stop…**

At this point the patient is probably thinking this is going to involve pain and discomfort so we need to reassure them we will do everything possible to keep them comfortable.

Explain that we have advanced technology that enables us to be incredibly effective in dealing with the bacteria, without pain.

I have found, the best analogy that help patients understand what needs to be done, is when I make a comparison with a splinter.

You can explain it's like having a splinter under the skin.

"If we don't get rid of the splinter you're never going to heal. In the same way, we need to do the cleaning to get the buildup out and to clear the area of bacteria".

If a patient has not been in for some time, this helps to explain why more action is needed, than a 'standard' cleaning. They need to catch up.

#2: *"We need to change a few things that you are doing at home."*

You have to be very careful here - It's been proven that nobody likes to get a lecture on what they are not doing.

So we need to position this carefully. We may suggest they use a prescription mouth wash daily to help keep the bacteria under control.

They are often open to this and people are willing to use what we recommend if they truly believe we believe it will help them.

It can also help to recommend using a power toothbrush.

When it comes to recommending the power brush, I often use the analogy of a screwdriver – a basic job can be done with a manual screwdriver but a big job will need a power screwdriver.

With the level of infection they have in their mouth, it requires a tool that will do more for them.

"In the same way, the infection that has built up in your mouth means you need a power brush to get rid of it. We need something that can do more for you than a basic manual toothbrush."

When introducing the idea of a power brush, it can be useful to say:

"We don't care where you get it as long as you get one."

You can suggest that high-end brushes such as Sonicare, or Oral B have been found to be more effective than manual brushing and add:

"We carry them, here in the office, because we know you are busy and we try to make everything as easy for you as possible. Plus, we can provide them for you at a cost less than you would pay at Wal-Mart."

The patient then understands we're not just trying to push a sale; we're trying to give them the tools they need to be more effective against the infection.

#3: *"We need to see you back more often."*

We know how important it is for the patients to come in for three or four-month recall visits but patients don't realize how critical it is. They are only used to hearing that they need to have their teeth cleaned every 6 months.

They don't know that bacteria has been proven to regenerate in just 21-60 days after scaling and root planing – and that they can have re-infection and more bleeding, within that time.

Patients really appreciate when we simplify things for them so it often helps to use the 'oil change' analogy.

We explain that after the deep cleaning, they are starting with a clean slate but if they don't come back more often – they may end up back where they started.

If we don't remain vigilant the disease will flare up. This disease will always remain, we MUST maintain it. Much like diabetes, it will always need maintenance.

We explain that it's like buying a brand new car – it won't last very long if you don't change the oil regularly.

So, to maximize healing, we need to see them back more often than they may have come in the past.

The latest research helps us to understand that maximizing our role as a periodontal therapist is not just about saving teeth, it really is about saving lives.

We know that dental health affects overall health but patients do not. There's compelling scientific proof that dental health affects overall health – for example people with periodontal disease are at greater risk of heart disease.

The National Institute of Health states,

"Oral bacteria shed from chronic periodontal infections enter the circulatory system and may contribute to diseases of the heart and other organs.

The role of periodontal diseases in causing or contributing to other serious conditions is the subject of ongoing laboratory and clinical research.

As this research unfolds in the coming years, it may be that a trip to the dentist not only could have benefits for your oral health but also help reduce your chances of developing related systemic conditions."

Scientists now know that the bacteria in our mouths exist as a complex, multi-layered community called oral biofilm.

Scientists already are in the process of dissecting the dynamics of these bacterial communities. This research may give dentists and hygienists the tools to target their treatment specifically to the bacteria that trigger periodontal disease.

We are already seeing this with laser procedures specifically targeting diseased tissues.

This is why for us to truly maximize our role as a periodontal therapist, we need constant refreshers. We MUST keep our protocol, and our techniques up to date in this critical area.

If you haven't embraced new technology or made any critical changes to your periodontal program in a few years, it is time to take a hard look at doing this now.

CHAPTER 5

How To Maximize The Patient Treatment Advocate

The third role is that of a Patient Treatment Advocate. Hygienists often underestimate what a critical role we have in helping our patients make choices about the dentistry they need.

How many times have they turned to the hygienist, or another clinical team member to ask, "Do I really need to have this done?" or "How long can I wait before I get this taken care of?"

The reality is, patients do want the team's opinion, and recommendations when it comes to the choices they have about treatment.

Did you know that 65% of all production completed in the Restorative Department in a dental practice is referred from hygiene?

If this is true, I often wonder why so many dentists feel like they could use more personal help in this area.

What tools do you have for aiding you in Case presentation?

Are you consistently using them?

How involved is the hygiene team in this effort?

The old paradigm for Case Presentation is to educate, educate, educate. Although I do think educating the patient is important, we have to remember to keep things simple.

When we use complicated terminology, the patient often ends up being confused. This is the last thing we want! Confused patients are unable to make a decision about treatment.

Do you ever hear, "I want to get it taken care of, but I need to go home and check with my spouse."

Patients needing to check their schedules call their insurance, or any other number of excuses, are most likely confused about recommendations, overwhelmed or both!

This leads to frustration. These 3 emotions are usually behind case acceptance failures and we must avoid them at all costs: Confusion, Overwhelm and Frustration.

Our challenge then is to approach Case presentation with the new paradigm. I have several key rules that if followed can help you explode your Case Acceptance.

Rule #1: Simplify! Talk in terms your patients understand. Often it's not what you say, but how you say it. In Case Acceptance, what THEY SEE is so much more important than what YOU SAY!

This is why I love to use my tools! There are several things I can't live without when talking with patients about opportunity for treatment in their mouths.

- Diagnodent, or as the patients know it, the "Cavity Detecting Laser" helps patients see things for themselves. They hear the alarm signal, they see the number (I have the patient hold it so they can participate) and they know without me having to say anything that there is a potential problem. Follow this up with another powerful tool, your intra-oral camera. Show them exactly what that reading of 34 looks like and why you are concerned.

- Intra-Oral Camera, again the value of this tool is that the patients can see for themselves. A cracked tooth in the mouth, and a cracked tooth up on the monitor or television look like two different things. I prefer my patients see it as big as life on the screen. This way, there is urgency without me having to create it for them.. The images from the camera take away any doubts the patient may have about their mouth.

"Seeing is Believing" is what it's all about!

Comments from the patient prove how powerful the camera is. I can't tell the patient that their teeth look terrible, but once they see it with the camera, often they are the ones that will say, "It looks terrible!"

Many practices have these amazing tools, but they sit collecting dust.

Lack of systems, perception that there "just isn't enough time" or lack of confidence on the part of the hygiene team often are the cause of underutilized valuable resources.

In reality, once hygienists learn that properly using these tools, and presenting opportunities with the right verbal skills actually SAVES time.

If you want more success with case acceptance, dust off the Diagnodent, take out that camera and get going!

Rule #2- Build Value - Patients will find a way to pay for what they WANT. So we should really focus on helping them want to have their teeth taken care of.

Why should they want to have this done?

Why would YOU do it?

Talk about this with your patients! I often will say, if this was in my mouth, this is what I would do to fix it. They are looking to us for guidance. They value and want out opinion.

So, to be more effective when talking with patients about what they need, don't be afraid to tell them what you would do. We should focus more often on what the direct benefits are.

Instead of telling the patient how we place implants, tell them the benefits of having them.

"When we place implants in your mouth, you will be able to chew without pain, almost like natural teeth. There will be nothing to take out and clean, you will be able to brush and floss these teeth as you did before. By the way, have I told you that implants have porcelain crowns on them that look incredibly like natural teeth?"

Building Value while keeping things simple can revolutionize your acceptance. Avoid the natural tendency to make things too complicated. Focus on the benefits for the patient, and they will be interested in learning more.

You will be amazed at what your patients accept when they understand what you are recommending, and WANT to have it done!

CHAPTER 6

How To Conduct An Effective New Patient Exam in 8 Minutes Or Less

By Dr. John Meis

What I learned most from my medical scare was that my practice and my family were not prepared to live without me. And that scared me straight.

I was determined to figure out HOW I could turn my little practice in Sioux City Iowa into financial security as quickly as humanly possible.

What follows is exactly what I did to raise my personal productivity to over $225,000 a month and place my practice and myself in the top 1% nationally. Over a 4 year time period (following this system) I was able to triple my practice.

How to Maximize The Clinical Production

While we are maximizing every part of our hygiene production, there are quite a few things that can be done to maximize the clinical production at the same time.

Here are the 5 major areas that I look at:

1. The Efficient and Effective New Patient Exam:
2. Clear Diagnostic Criteria (Tribal Language):
3. Maximizing Same Day Dentistry
4. Increasing the Toolbelt
5. Case Presentation

The Efficient and Effective New Patient Exam

There are still quite a few practices that are still practicing with out of date information, and it's hurting your productivity and profitability.

The new patient exam is a place where I see this more often than not. Doctors are still wanting long exam times, patient education only done by the doctor, collecting vast data on every patient whether there is any clinical reason or not. Many still want one diagnostic visit and a separate case presentation visit.

While all the above was great, the more information we had gathered, the better informed we could be, but this is ...

Not what our patients want

Patients want effective and efficient exams. And it's not just the exam – they want effective and efficient dental visits.

When the patient has an immediate problem, and they have come in to have that problem fixed. The doctor can do a limited exam on that one problem only, solve that problem or if they can't solve the problem today, schedule them for the solution.

There is no reason why a comprehensive exam couldn't be done at the same time.

One of the best indicators of profitability for your practice is your comprehensive to limited exam ratio.

This ratio will also tell us how much opportunity currently exists in your practice.

What should your ratio be?

For a mature practice – it should be at least 60% comprehensive. For a younger practice it should be higher.

The first 'sale' for a new patient should be the 'sale' into a comprehensive exam, whether that's what the patient came in for or not.

The #1 Reason Given

I've learned that "I can't afford it" is the #1 reason given when any patient is presented with the comprehensive exam (when it's not what they came in for.)

But I have also learned that people will say they can't afford things that they can afford and they do it all the time.

So, why is it the answer that we hear all the time? Most do it because they don't want to give you the less polite answer. Most don't want to tell you that your office is dirty, or your staff is rude, or they don't feel comfortable in your practice.

They say they can't afford it. It's just an easy way to get out without having some socially awkward conversation.

Most doctors would say… well, if they can't afford the exam, they can't afford the treatment, so why should I waste my time?

WRONG. If this is the response in your office, or worse yet amongst your staff … you are letting money walk right out your back door day in and day out.

One of the things that I would do, when I heard this, is

to say

> *"Well that's all right, but why don't we do this… Why don't I pay for your exam and x-rays, and that way you can see what's going on in your mouth and have a better idea of how to go about fixing it."*

I realized that sometimes (many times) money was just an excuse, often an excuse because they were fearful. If the money was the real objection, I had solved it. If the money wasn't the real objection, this helped me bring the real objection to the surface so I could handle it.

I found very frequently that the objection was that the patient was fearful and we weren't managing their anxiety properly.

Effective Exams

Let's talk about being effective first… It all starts with an introduction from the team.

I'll talk more about the team's role here in just a bit…. But let's start with when you walk through the door.

You want the patient to be sitting up, so you can sit down <u>in front</u> (not behind, not off to the side, but in front) of the patient, eye-to-eye, knee-to-knee, introduce yourself and prepare to receive the hand-off from your team.

I've been in, over 150 different dental practices across North America. One of the things that I have seen surprisingly frequently is that doctor comes in and they first start to look at something. They look at the new patient form, they look at the x-rays. They make no connection with the patient immediately.

From the patients perspective this is extremely awkward, and I understand what the doctor is trying to do. They're trying to get a sense of the situation before they talk with the patients. But it's just so awkward and deters from the patient experience.

Introduce yourself, sit facing the patient so that they can see you, and SMILE. After you've introduced yourself, it's time for the hand-off.

The hand-off from your team should include all of the information that has been gathered already, and when done properly, creates a tremendous amount of efficiency and allows us to keep the new patient exam in under 8 minutes. When the hand-off is done improperly it creates 2x the amount of work, and takes 2x as long.

Immediately following the hand-off, you want to make an emotional connection with your patient.

The Untold Key To High Case Acceptance: The EMOTIONALLY CONNECTED Exam

The first thing to do is to stop and avoid the connection stoppers. There are three of them that I see all of the time:

1. Judging
2. Shaming
3. Indifference

The secret is through an emotionally connected exam and the only way to do that is to emotionally connect with your patient.

Either you the doctor, or your team that has seen the patient before you needs to identify what the dominant emotion is of that patient.

Are they worried?

Are they anxious?

Are they angry?

What are they feeling?

Once you identify what that dominant emotion is you need to relate to that. I've seen a lot of dentists and I've watched a lot of new patient exams. I watch where a new patient will tell the doctor that they're scared and the dentist just goes right past it.

Or they will tell the doctor that they're upset with their last dentist and the doctor avoids it like it was a hot rock and they didn't want to touch it.

But on the other side, from the patient's perspective,

the doctor seems to be indifferent… he seems to not care.

One of the things people are looking for in a provider is somebody who cares. You have to relate to that emotion.

So, how can we relate?

You can say something like, "Tell me more about that," or "How so?" As they begin to talk more and open up more, you start getting a sense of what they're looking for by relating to that emotion.

Something has caused that emotion, and once you know what that emotion is, you can adapt to it, and most importantly you can say it out loud to the patient.

If a patient said to me… "I'm afraid of needles" I would respond back *so you would really like to lessen or eliminate the experience with needles, is that right?*

They of course would say yes. Now they're getting the understanding that I am listening and I am tuning in and I am trying to give them what they want.

Once they tell me that I'm on the right track, I would say, "*What else would you like?*", or "*What else would you like to avoid?*"

Once I've really followed this down the path as far as I can go, then I summarize it.

I say, "*You would like to have x, y and z? You'd like to avoid, a, b, c? Do I have that right?"* Then, again, I listen to the patient, if they add something to it I hadn't gone far enough.

This is the part of the exam for me that actually takes the biggest single section of time, making sure that I understand where they are **emotionally**, that I've connected with it and I've addressed it in a way that they are satisfied with.

If you fail to make an emotional connection, your case acceptance is going to be much lower than it needs to be.

The Efficient Exam

Let's talk about the exam and being efficient. In order to be highly efficient, we as the doctor, have to give up what feels like our control in the situation.

Where most people fail, is they blindly give up control. I believe that you should maintain your control but give up the need to do everything yourself.

The only way to do this successfully is to create systems and train your team on your philosophies, and thought processes.

To start, **the team gathers all data**. Assistants or hygienists will gather the following:

- Radiographs
- Intra-oral photos

- Study models (if needed)
- Face-bow (if needed)
- Bite registration (if needed)

The hygienist will do the perio exam, and pre-assess, what they think is a reasonable treatment plan. In addition, they will educate the patient on periodontal disease.

The goal is to have your team understand your treatment planning philosophy and your treatment planning criteria so well that they have a very good understanding of what the case is (more on this in the next chapter.) With this, they can now begin to discuss potential treatment needs and educate the patient on those needs.

For instance, a team member might say something like,

> *"Well I'm not the doctor and we'll need to talk to him or her. But in the past he or she has... when they've seen this kind of condition has recommended this, let me tell you about it."*

So that when the doctor hits the door, the patient understands largely what their treatment needs are going to be, and they understand what those treatments are.

When the doctor does hit the door, he does what I talked about already; he introduces himself, creates an emotional connection, and then receives the hand-off from the team member.

These are some elements of a good hand-off (and you will need to work out the elements that work for you):

- I always like to know the patient's name and how to pronounce it correctly.

- I want to know something personal about that patient. If the team member has found something personal that is a common interest of mine, that's even more helpful because now we can have something to bond on.

- Then hopefully the staff member has already identified what the dominant emotion is. They may not have gone down into the path like I described earlier, but they hopefully will be able to tell you at least what that dominant emotion was done.

- The team member then tells you what was done, what data was gathered, and what was discussed. What conditions were discussed? What treatments were discussed?

For me, that was an outstanding hand-off. Very, very rarely do I see this from team members in the practices that I visit.

What I usually see is, the Doctor comes in, staff has a lot of information but they don't share it with the doctor. The doctor's flying blind and it <u>takes more time</u>.

That added time doesn't provide any value to the

patient. In fact, it decreases value to the patient. Because now, the patient is covering things with the doctor that they have already covered with the team member.

After the hand-off, the doctor proceeds to do his exam (both extro-oral and intra-oral), reviews the radiographs, and for most patients, a treatment plan and a presentation can be done.

I understand that a treatment plan and presentation can not be done immediately in every case, but its usually only 10% of the time it when it can't be.

Times when there are severe wear cases, severe plane of occlusion problems, severely unstable TMJ joints, implant cases where you're not sure if there's enough bone and you need additional radiography like a cone beam. These are all the exceptions. But really they're not more than 10% of the cases, 90% of the time you can move right into the treatment plan and presentation.

First we're going to focus on what the patient wants because the team has already figured that out exactly what the patient wants.

In your discussion with them, the emotional connection, you already know what they want, and can focus first on that.

Then discuss what they need, identify where they would like to start.

One of the best ways I saw this presented was in

talking about neighborhoods in the mouth. If the patient was drawn to the office because they had a problem in the lower right, you talk about taking care of everything on the lower right by saying, "there are other neighborhoods to take care of but would you like to start here?"

The next thing you need to do is to create urgency and show that this needs to be done now. You need put a time frame on it.

IF you don't create urgency patients don't think it's important.

CHAPTER 7

How To Increase Case Acceptance Using Tribal Language

By Dr. John Meis

Clear Diagnostic Criteria: What I have seen is very scary... if you were to show the same patient to 10 different dentists, you will likely receive a range of treatment plans from the most productive to the least productive based on each Dentists' subjective data and personal treatment planning.

This is not good, especially when the range of treatment is occurring in one office.

Dentistry isn't black and white. Which means that it is your responsibility to define the diagnostic and treatment criteria for your practice.

Not only will each dentist have a different opinion on the treatment plan for our patient, if you were to ask each doctor at different times of the day for their diagnoses, you would again have a range of answers.

When we are fresh (IE in the morning), we tend to be more aggressive in our treatment recommendations and we are fired up to utilize our same day dentistry skills. As the day wears on, our treatment planning may become a little more conservative… we are willing to 'wait' on some things that we might not have put off in the morning.

Because of this, your practice needs to have criteria set in place based on where you, the doctor, feel most comfortable treating your patients.

You need to define things like;

1. What defines a cavity mean in your practice? …. What are the radiographic findings that indicate decay?

2. What are the criteria for determining that crown is needed? What are the clinical findings that indicate that a filling will no longer work?

3. What are the symptoms that indicate that endo is needed?

4. When is a tooth damaged beyond repair?

5. Which tooth replacement is ideal?

6. When do we use a removable prosthesis to replace the teeth?

7. When do we use a fixed prosthesis supported by teeth or implants?

8. When do we use a removable that's supported by teeth implants and/or tissue?

When you have your criteria spelled out and defined you have a standard of measurement to ensure that you are not over-diagnosing and not-under-diagnosing AND more importantly, you can now utilize your entire team in presenting treatment.

Without defined criteria, you will have varying levels of care for your patients depending on which provider they saw that day. This only increases the patients level of confusion.

We want to be crystal clear and ensure that every provider and every team member that they see that day is able to provide the patient with the reassurance that the recommended treatment is the best course of treatment.

This can only be accomplished if the entire team has defined criteria and uses the same language.

We accomplish this 'across team' communication by using what we call 'Tribal Language.' We have found that everything we defined above, can be placed into 3 categories:

1. **Mandatory:** these are the most urgent needs, and are for problems that involve anything that is broken, infected or decayed. This is the building is on fire, and we need to get the fire out

2. **Elective:** is something that can cause a future problem if not addressed at some point. This is what used to be our 'watch' list.

3. **Cosmetic:** is something that would cosmetically enhance the appearance of the smile.

This also provides the patient with a clear picture and allows the patient to direct their course of treatment and be in control of their treatment

I took an evening, to place all of my criteria into these 3 categories, using the worksheet pictured. I then laminated this and placed it in our team room and every operatory, so that everyone had access to our team's tribal language.

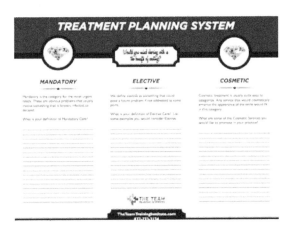

As the hygienist are utilizing their 3 roles, they start this process by speaking in this language. And are pre-warming the patient so that when you come in and present your treatment they are open to the idea.

> **To download this worksheet and the definitions to create Mandatory/Elective/Cosmetic language in your practice go to:**
>
> **www.TheTeamTrainingInstitute.com/M-E-C**

Having your team pre-assess using your diagnostic criteria is not only helpful, but becomes a critical and often overlooked step in the case presentation and case acceptance. This is the piece of the puzzle that allows for same-day-dentistry.

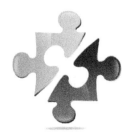

CHAPTER 8

The Secret To Creating RAVING Fans And Increased Production

By Dr. John Meis

I think that Zig Zigler said it best... *"You can have everything you want in life, if you will just help enough people get what they want."*

What is it that our patient wants? They want to have everything taken care of in one visit. They don't want to have to come back in. So how do we give them what they want?

Same Day Dentistry

When provided effectively this is THE biggest

contributor to patients RAVING about your practice. It's simply providing the patients with what they want most – an effective dental visit, where everything is taken care of and they don't have to schedule another appointment. It's HIGHLY convenient and improves productivity dramatically.

In a recent survey from 1-800 dentists, patients stated that the having a CONVENIENT Dentist is the second most important thing to them (the #1 thing that they want is a clear and honest explanation about costs.)

What is same-day-dentistry?

It simply means that when we diagnose or find an opportunity for continued care, we offer the patient the opportunity to accept that treatment today and not have to schedule and come in for another appointment. <u>It is dentistry that was completed today that was not on the schedule this morning.</u>

In the past, if it wasn't on the schedule to be treated today, it meant another appointment.

If you wanted sealants – you scheduled another appointment.

If there was a small cavity – you scheduled another appointment.

If you had a root canal it was another 3 appointments!

What can be done with Same Day Dentistry:

- ➢ Emergency Call-In Patients – "How soon can you get here?"

- ➢ Converting New Patients from a limited to a comprehensive exam

- ➢ Treatment diagnosed today

- ➢ Restorative work scheduled... "while you are here and numb in this area, should we also take care of...?"

- ➢ Hygiene Patients … previously diagnosed and uncompleted treatment, newly diagnosed treatment and preventative services

The best part … no one can cancel the appointment because they are already there ☺

But, I don't have TIME to do this

I am sure that you are shaking your head going, "…sure that all sounds great in theory…but we are barely getting everything done that we need to get done. There is no way that I can add more to the plate."

And I 100% agree with you, you can't add anything more to the plate doing what you currently do.

Today is the day that you need to commit to changing the way that you currently operate. In chapter 3, 4, & 5, that is what we asked of your hygienists, and now it's your turn.

I promise, it's not difficult, in fact it wasn't that long ago that I made these changes to my practice. When I did … my practice tripled in the next 4 years!

What do you need to do to prepare and offer same-day-dentistry:

Every Room Is Identical

A big reason that you are not able to add anything more to your current schedule is because you have maxed out your way of scheduling and utilizing your operatories.

I will make a bet, that Susie only uses op 4 and Vicky is always in op 6 and if I was wagering, I would also say they look a lot like this -------→

To best utilize every inch of your practice and every minute of your day, you will need to un-nest your rooms. When someone feels like an operatory is 'theirs' they tend to move-in.

There are pictures of their family, personal items, in some practices their name is even on the wall.

This limits you to who can use this room and when they can use it.

So we have every room equipped identically. Every door has the same thing. Everything is exactly the same from room-to-room, to the degree that it can be.

No nesting, team members don't have "their" room. There isn't a room called Sally's room or Susie's room, that's room 1, that's room 2, because Susie and Sally will be working in more than one room. They will be moving around the office as necessary while same day treatment is being done

Is every operatory room in your practice equipped identically? Is everything located in the same place in each room? When it's not equipped and supplied the same our ops become less efficient and our production becomes less efficient.

This is the key to being able to practice in any open exam room…. which is the key to maximizing same-day-dentistry.

Why would we do this? Because it's more convenient for the patient to remain in one room and have the team move around, AND this is the way to maximize your schedule.

Having enough team members

Generally, the minimum number of dental assistants

that a practice should have is the number of rooms minus the number of hygienists.

In other words if there's a room, it should have an assistant. A room without an assistant isn't very valuable.

Have enough rooms

You will know when you start to run out, because you'll have treatment that could be done and you don't have a room to do it in.

That should never ever, ever, ever happen. You should always have another room to do another procedure.

This is the most common piece to the same-day-dentistry puzzle – running out of rooms. You can get more rooms. You can add rooms.

You can do it by eliminating a doctor office, the break room, a conference room, any extra rooms.

I had one practice that had a workout room in their building. They eliminated their workout room and added more ops.

Standard ops are usually somewhere between 12 and 16-feet wide. But if the room is designed properly you can actually have an op in a space less 9-feet wide.

The 2-for-3 switch, was designed by Dr. David Ahern, and involves taking two rooms into three. It works exceedingly well when a practice cannot move their four walls and doesn't have any other space that can be turned into ops.

If after you have exhausted all of your options to increase your room space, the next thing option, is to expand hours.

Expanding hours doesn't make sense if you only have one doctor provider. If you're going to extend hours, it means expanding doctor providers, which we'll talk about in a later chapter.

After that, the next way to get additional rooms is having a new and different or additional facility.

Bonus the Team

Another thing that helps same-day-dentistry is to bonus the team.

If a team member identifies a same day opportunity, they get a bonus and the team member that accepts taking care of the patient during that same-day opportunity gets a bonus.

I see practices that do bonuses of $5 each person, per each event. I've seen practices do as much as $15, but I feel that $5 is often enough.

Have a Clinical Coordinator

The last of the same-day tips, if the practice is big enough, usually more than 8 operatories, having a clinical coordinator is very helpful. A clinical coordinator is often the traffic cop.

They're watching the schedule, they know who is where, what team member is where, and when a room might be open.

They're stepping in to help with sterilization, or room turnover or assisting if needed. They're the person making sure that everything is running smoothly in the practice and that we're capturing every single same-day opportunity that we can.

Just because you have built a practice that can accommodate same-day-dentistry doesn't mean they will come.

Like all presentations in Dentistry, there is a wrong way and a right way to present options for same-day-dentistry.

Here are a few questions to start driving your same-day-dentistry:

- If possible, would you like to get this taken care of today?

- It might mean a little bit of a wait, is that OK?

- Do you have a preference which doctor you see, or would you like the first available doctor?

CHAPTER 9

Increase Your Toolbelt Increase Your Profits

By Dr. John Meis

Every time that you refer a patient out your door, you are losing potential production that could have been kept in house. In the next chapters, I will show you how you can free up more of your time to be spent on higher productive dental work.

Are You Letting Profits Walk Right Out Your Door?

You should be doing everything possible to increase the tools in your toolbelt and reduce the amount of work that you need to refer out.

I became certified and trained to do my own endo, sedation, implants, cosmetic dentistry, and surgery AND my practice COULD NOT have tripled without these skills.

When I left dental school, I was NOT comfortable doing anything but your basic drilling and filling. So, I had to put in time and money to better those skills.

And the pay off …. Well, my practice tripled in production and I was personally in the top 1% of all producers.

Now, the only things that I refer out are the particularly complex and difficult cases that need a specialist.

I used to think that my patients wanted to go to see a specialist for everything.

What I found, was that I was the one who had established a rapport and connection with my patients and they were much more comfortable having me do as much dentistry as possible.

They didn't want to have to make an appointment with a strange doctor, if the doctor that they knew, liked and trusted could take care of it for them.

Confident Case Presentation

The one area that is most critical for Dentists to master is case presentation. The financial future of your practice and your family becomes solely reliant on this skill.

And that is exactly what it is… a skill. Something that you need to learn and practice to excel at.

It is also the one place where most Dentists shy away from. They do everything possible to avoid having to ask the patient for money. I don't want you to think about it like that.

Your job is to UNDERSTAND what your patients WANT, understand what your patients NEED and then negotiate for optimal treatment.

How do you do that?

By now, you have hopefully noticed that all of the skills and ideas that we have presented in this book are intertwined and run throughout your practice and throughout the patients experience with your practice.

Because, nothing happens in a vacuum.

If you want to become better at case presentation, it starts with the presentation of your office as a new patient walks through the door, actually it starts with the presentation in their first call to your office, their experience parking and entering your building.

Your patients are coming in with a particular WANT.

Mostly it's a dental related problem, but many severe problems are asymptomatic and patients aren't aware that they have a problem.

That is why … everything in the first few chapters is all about the Hygienists (our first line of providing dental care) advocating for the patient and working with the patient to UNDERSTAND what they want and to start the process of understanding what the NEEDS are, so that your case presentation job of negotiating for their optimal treatment becomes much easier.

If the Hygienists have done a good job, using their tools to showcase where the patients health currently stands, worked with the patient to understand their current wants, exposed possible areas (like de-sensitizing treatments and sealants) and they have introduced the tribal language and introduced what they are seeing as potential mandatory – elective – and cosmetic options, and educated the patient. When you come in, the patient will likely have an expanded view of what they want, from when they first walked in the door.

What this really comes down to is having a good way to communicate with patients about what they need.

First, understanding what they want, and then helping them understand what they need and having a dialogue to determine what ultimately should be done.

I typically present either in an operatory or in a separate consult room. It worked fine for me to do it in the op, which means a little more efficiency with my time (and the patients, since there is no moving).

When I am in the op, the patient is sitting up. Again, we're eye-to eye, knee-to-knee and I'm discussing what my findings are.

If I do it in a consult room, I prefer not to sit across a desk. I'd rather come around, sit in the same type of chair. I don't want to have a big fancy executive chair that I'm wheeling around in. I want the patient and I to be a team of equals dealing with the issues that they have.

Confident Case Presentation

Confidence draws people in, people tend to listen to confident people and dismiss those that lack confidence. Here are a couple of ways that you can appear confident:

#1: Provide few options. Be confident in your decision and provide a best choice first and a less expensive (and less, from a patient's perspective less quality) as a second option. And then stop talking.

For instance, if we are talking about tooth replacement, I would offer a permanent option that doesn't come in and out of their mouth as their best option, and something that is removable as a secondary option.

#2: Using wishy-washy or minimizing language. Wishy-washy is:

"Well maybe we could do this" or

"maybe we could try this" or
"this most likely will work"

I understand that we can't guarantee anything, patients are biological creatures and biological creatures are by their nature unpredictable, BUT

When you communicate that way, it comes across to the patient as you not being confident. Patients are looking for confidence from their health care providers.

The other way I see is using minimizing language:

"It's a little cavity"
"It's a minor infection"
"It's this or it's that."

With words that make it seem not serious and not urgent. That just kills a patient's drive to get it taken care of.

One of the best ways to show your confidence is to represent the recommendation that you're giving them as the same one that you would give to a loved one.

For instance, *"if you were my mother, this is what I would be recommending for you."*

Make sure you are using age and gender appropriate comparisons. You wouldn't say to a man, "if you were my mother, I would do this" (I never know if someone is taking my words literally ☺)

I always err on the side of caution, If the woman is just old enough to be my mother, I would saying, *"if you were my sister,"* always use the younger age comparison, not dramatically younger but younger.

You always want to presume that they're younger than they are. (Save yourself a lot of insult and grief).

What Doesn't Work - Long explanations.: I see dentists willing to talk about what's wrong, willing to talk about what can be done about it. Then they talk forever <u>about how it's done.</u>

Patients don't care about how it's done (a handful might, but the vast majority won't.) What they do care about is how this will change their life and what will happen if they don't fix it.

What Does Work: You want to have a short explanation that describes what's wrong, what can be done about it, and what will happen if they don't do it.

What If I Use A Treatment Coordinator To Close My Cases?

The position of treatment coordinator is different in different practices. The way I look at, it's anyone who is handling or 'closing the case.'

They are talking about the treatment and the financial arrangements. They are the ones who are doing the scheduling. They're getting the patient to commit.

I found it helpful to have this person in the room for the exam and case presentation. You need to make sure that any person in this role has an understanding of dentistry as well as an understanding of financial arrangements.

Their job is to help the patient afford the treatments. They have to understand the financial options, and we like to present those options as a ladder.

The first step is what's best for the patient and the practice. That's cash. We offer a cash discount if they pre-pay for their care.

We then move then to a credit card option.

Then we talk about support from families, or anybody they know that would be able help with the treatment or that would be willing to help with the treatment?

Then we go to third party financing. Once we are at third party financing, we talk about a family member or friend being a co-signer for the third-party financing.

If we haven't found a solution yet, we start to break the treatment into quadrants or less, so we reduce the amount of treatment being done.

As a last resort, we would change from the more natural, more comfortable, and more long-lasting restoration to one that's less natural but less expensive.

PART 2

Systematize for Success

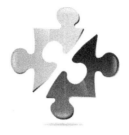

CHAPTER 10

How To Systematize Your Practice

By Dr. John Meis

Step #2: Create Systems for staff, space, and equipment

There is a point, and for you I am guessing you are at this point or you wouldn't have found us, that the cobbled together 'systems' in your practice can no longer support your growth… you need to create true systems (meaning they will work regardless of who you put in the practice) to give you, the doctor, time to actually do the Dentistry!

Your outstanding office manager is at their wits end just trying to keep their head above water and shudder each time you mention "we need more new patients" or needing to increase revenue.

The biggest mistake most people make is that they go about creating training for their team members and not enough systems.... If you are currently relying on the talent of your team members instead of the talent of your system, you are at risk when your talented team member leaves.

Unfortunately, there will never be a time when you are assured 100% that one of your team members won't leave. That is why it is necessary to create a system that will allow you to plug a new team member in and build your talent within your system.

I knew a practice that had a very talented person doing their financial arrangements. We used to joke that she could get homeless people to buy expensive dentistry.

She was extremely talented, but there were no systems. The practice relied on her great talent. And then she left...

The practice began to struggle. And it took them several years to get back to where they were. They had to start by creating a system.

The thing to remember is ... great systems endure, talented people don't always.

Systems allow for better delegation. They provide for more treatment to be done and they save doctor time.

They save your mental energy as well. As health care providers, we run out of mental energy before we run out of physical energy.

What happened when I first implemented systems in my practice?

At one time, I was running all the meetings. Once a system was in place, others could lead those meetings ... here's what that meant to me.

I know that good meetings require significant preparation time. It takes me about three times the length of the meeting to prep for a meeting when I'm going to be doing all the presentations.

My practice started every morning with a 15-minute huddle, we also had one weekly one-hour meeting.

So, having someone else that was running the meetings and the preparation, saved a tremendous amount of time.

Fifteen-minute huddle x 5 days a week x three = That's 225 minutes a week in prep time that I didn't have to do.

Prepping for the one-hour team meeting meant another 180 minutes.

Altogether having someone take over this and follow the system that was created saved me 6.75 hours a week!

My production, at the time, was about $1300 an hour, so 6.75 extra hours now spent producing dentistry, meant an extra $8,800 per week in production.

Do you get it?

When I transitioned the time I was spending prepping for meeting into production, my production would go up $8,800 per week.

The end-result of this one system was we had better meetings, because I hadn't been doing the amount of prep that I should have, and we ended up having better trained teams because the meetings were so much more educational when they were given appropriate preparation.

We were much better organized and it improved the patient experience dramatically and it increased production.

This one system just on the timesaving's, created an additional $440,000 per year of production for our practice.

That's an example of what just one system can do to increase your production! Imagine what can happen when you implement multiple systems ☺

But in order to do this and to add in everything that we recognized in step #1 we can no longer do what we were doing and expect different results (in fact wanting that.... To keep doing the same things over and over again and expecting different results is actually the true definition of insanity)

Warning: Most practices THINK that they have a system ... but a system is defined as having 4 components:

1. Commanders' Intent: Why is this important and what is the purpose of this system

2. Flow Chart: Showing the different steps of the system and who is responsible for each step.

3. Scripts: Define the communication expected, examples of any media that might help

4. Follow-up Mechanism: to create checks and balances and ensure that the system is implemented. These need to be a part of the daily/weekly/monthly routine.

So what should you have a system for:

Operations:

- Effective Meetings
- Morning Huddles
- Internal Marketing Strategies
- External Marketing
- Patient Attraction
- Emotionally Connected New Patient Exam
- New Patient Experience
- Confident Case Presentation
- Perio-Case Acceptance
- Tribal Language
- Patient Friendly Financials
- Scheduling for Success
- Recall, Recovery, Reactivation, Retention and Referrals

- Insurance Billing
- Room Set Up
- Same-Day-Dentistry
- Children's Programs
- Home Products
- Cancellations
- Monthly Financials
- Accounts Receivable
- Front Desk Check-in
- Seamless Handoffs
- System Sterilization

Clinical Procedures:

- Perio-Health Maintenance
- 6-Point Probing
- Hygiene Services: Fluoride, Sealant, De-sensitizing Treatment, & Radiograph Protocols
- Crown & Bridge Protocol
- Sedation Protocol
- Root Canal Protocol
- Caries Detection Protocol
- Risk Assessment Protocol
- Intraoral Camera Protocol
- Diagnostic Code
- Clinical Note & Charting and Documentation Protocol
- Cavity Detecting Laser Protocol
- Oral Cancer Screening Protocol

- World-Class Exam Protocol

Human Resources:
- Hiring
- Firing
- Payroll
- 3/3/3 Training
- Personal Development Interviews
- Performance Reviews
- Bonus Systems

THE MOST IMPORTANT: A System for Creating Your Systems ☺

As you create each of these WRITTEN systems, you place them into a binder that all team members have access to.

Now, when a new team member starts, they follow the binder as a training mechanism.

This reduces the amount of time it takes to train a new team member, while keeping the entire team (including the doctor) accountable for the metrics that you have set forth.

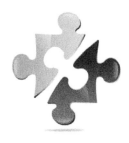

CHAPTER 11

How To Build A Leadership Team To Support Your Growth

By Dr. John Meis

Step #3: Build a Leadership Team

Does this sound familiar?

You are running around the practice, like a chicken with their head cut off, answering a question for the front desk staff about your schedule, then you move to the assistant wanting to know if you can do a check in exam room 2, but Susie needs to know if you wanted all 3 sizes of the gloves or if we only need mediums this month, you have a hygienist wanting to set up an interview for the open position, and to top it all off your spouse calls to remind you that tonight you have parent teacher conferences and you need to be home no later than 5:45pm.

It's not even 9:30, you have only seen your first patient and you already feel exhausted.

Who Actually Handles The Practice Management?

I will bet you any amount of money, that you don't have a management team. Which means that you have to do everything yourself.

I know… you are a small practice, you can handle it all yourself….

But what you don't know, is that all of this is draining your mental energy and taking you away from what you are HIGHLY trained and skilled to do – practice dentistry.

Instead you are spending your day dealing with staff issues, marketing issues, following up to ensure that all the systems from chapter 10 are being created.

You are conducting all the team trainings, doing all the hiring, doing all the firing, doing the accounting and bookkeeping.

YOU DON'T HAVE TO BE THE ONLY ONE

When you are doing all of this, it is impossible to be

productive. The most productive dentists in the world don't do any of the above. They focus all their mental energy on creating the vision and goals for the practice, treating their patients, and safeguarding the money.

Everything else is delegated to somebody else because it can be.

If you have read any books on time management, one of the key strategies is to determine what your time is worth.

Take the amount of money that you made last year and divide it by the number of hours that you work. For simplicities sake, let's assume you brought home $100,000 last year and you worked the full 8 hours a day/5 days a week/ for 52 weeks a year (use 2,080).

So you will divide $100,000/2080 and you come up with $48.08. That is your hourly wage.

$200,000/year = $96.15/hour

$300,000/year = $144.23/hour

$500,000/year = $240.38/hour

You get the idea. Now that you have that number, I want you to write it down somewhere that you can refer back to it and next to it I want you to write what your average hourly production is as a doctor.

How Often Are You Losing Money?

Because every time you are doing a job, such as ordering supplies, or calling the newspaper about your marketing piece, or interviewing a hygienist – anything that you can hire someone to do for less per hour than you make, you are actually losing money.

Personally, I hate to do lawn-care. Heck, I can hire a kid to it for $20/week, which means that I can see one more patient at a billable rate of $1,750 during the time in which I used to be mowing the lawn.

What Can Be Delegated?

Here are just a few things on the clinical side;

- **Data gathering**, this can all be done by assistants or hygienists.

- **Documenting.** A doctor's role in documenting should be to read and review and make sure the documentation is correct. I see many doctors spending hours a day, doing charts, totally unnecessary. The documentation can be templated and the team can use the template and the doctor's responsibility is to review to make sure it's accurate. It saves hours of time everyday.

- Explaining **Treatment and Financial Options**. Both of these things can be done easily by other team members. It's unnecessary for the dentist to do.

- Depending on your state laws, **Taking Impressions, Making Temporaries, or even Placing Restorative Material**. Depending on the state you're in, anyone of those can be delegated to other team members.

Here are a few for the non-clinical side of your practice:

- Ordering supplies

- Taking care of the physical building; the lawn, the landscaping, the maintenance.

But I see doctors doing all of these and I see them doing it all the time. It just takes so much time that could be used to provide higher-value care for patients.

Now, I know you are already thinking… "But Dr. John, it's MY practice, if I am not looking after all of these things, we won't survive!"

You are right … and so am I ☺

You need to be LOOKING at the operations of your practice but not DOING the operations at your practice. Your job is to create a team of people around you who will DO - leaving you to simply follow up (utilizing about 1-2 hours a week of your time) with your team on their operation of your systems.

I know how hard it can be to let go of the control; after all you are talking to an OCD control freak here. But, once I learned this, my life and my practice were changed forever and I would never go back to the old way.

After all, do I really care what color the gloves are? Shouldn't I care more about knowing that we are working a system to ensure that we are never under or over stocked in any of our supplies?

See, once you have your SYSTEM in place, you can hire and develop a person to follow the system as you have designed it. You will quickly see that this process is what will give you and your team the confidence for growth.

It's scary to venture into the unknown – it's easier to stay with what you are comfortable with. But as I said before, if you continue doing what you are doing you will continue to get the same results.

When most people hear the word 'delegation,' they think that they are simply supposed to tell someone what they want done and then poof it's done. In the real world it never happens that way.

How Do You Actually Do This?

By developing a system based on the way that you want things to be done, and then training the person to follow the system, you ensure that things are being accomplished the way that you wanted....without you having to do it yourself.

OK, so now that we all agree that you need to create your systems, and we are in the chapter about creating a management team, so let's take a look at what that means…

The first thing that your management team will do is create and adhere to accountability. If you remember, we said at every system has a mechanism for accountability.

The management team isn't in charge of that accountability. They're in charge of seeing that the system is being followed and monitoring the results of the system.

What Does A Management Team Do?

If the results are not what we expect then they're coaching those using the system to attain the achievable results.

In addition, they're training new people on using the systems, and creating new systems. They're identifying places where things aren't working and creating systems to overcome those blockages.

I expect that these managers, will know their stuff, they'll know the services, and they'll **notice** when things aren't working. Their job is to notice when things aren't working.

They'll create new systems or improve the systems that exist to make them work more smoothly in every day practice life.

The Management team also does all the non-clinical things that the doctors are currently doing.

There are only 3 things that I DO NOT delegate and that ever Doctor should be looking at consistently

> **Strategic Planning**: You should have regular meeting with your clinic administrator to be strategically planning for the practices' future.

> **Accounting**: Theft in dental practices is way too common to delegate this or blindly let a team member be in full control of your money. The largest theft that occurred to someone I know, was almost $3 million embezzled from their practice.

  You need to be involved with this. You need to understand who's writing the checks and what they are writing the checks for. You need to understand your account adjustments very well.

> **Your Checkbook:** You need to understand who is balancing the checkbook and that should not be the same person who's writing the checks.

How My First Management Team Increased New Patients By 15%....And It Took NO TIME From Me

In looking at our data, I was able to determine that our new patient yield from new patient phone calls was low. *(side note: the only way I was able to know that this number was low was because I was a part of a group where I had benchmarks from practices that were doing better than we were)*

The management team created a system for answering the phone. They did training on it and they monitored it to make sure that the system was being followed.

We used a mechanism to create the ability to answer the phone more hours of the day and more days per week.

They created a bonus for every new patient scheduled; the team member who scheduled them would get a little bonus. In our practice that was $5 and it worked very well.

The result of this new system that the management team put in place was; a 15% increase in new patients.

Here's the beauty of it. <u>It took zero of my time.</u> That's what a management team can do.

All that took time, and without a management team, it would have come at the expense of my production.

Now, it all happened, it all was successful, and it took zero of my time

What Does This Look Like In A Practice?

The first management position that I put in a practice is that of a Clinic Administrator.

The Clinic Administrator is responsible for running all of the meetings and generally running the marketing systems. They are the ones who will handle the follow up and accountability for all of the systems designed (in Chapter 10)

They are the point person working the patient traction. They are watching the patient experience, looking for ways that they can improve the experience.

They become "HR," taking on the hiring and firing and other HR duties. They are ensuring that the practice is compliant with HIPPA, OSHA, and any other regulations. They are overseeing the training of new team members.

And this is an important one; they're constructively challenging the doctor. If the doctor is being the knucklehead, this is the person who has to tell him that he's being a knucklehead. Without this, doctors can get off-track.

Every doctor needs a clinic administrator where there is mutual respect and admiration, but also a little bit of an edge, as the clinic administrator's job is to drive the doctors. Keep them engaged, humble, and taking great care of patients.

When Do I Need A Clinic Administrator?

Let's look at what an ideal team should look like for your dental practice.

A Clinic Administrator can be implemented at any time, but if there are only 3-4 people in the practice, it might not be worth the time just yet.

Once a practice has between 5 and 9 team members, I would designate a clinic administrator (generally someone who also has front desk responsibilities).

For a practice that has more than 9 members, you have 2 choices, as the role of clinic administrator will be to challenging to do in addition to other practice duties.

Option 1: I would move the clinic administrator into a full time position (or hire for this position.)

Option 2: I would add an additional management role and I would have one administrative team leader and one clinical team leader.

At any point that you have more than 3 hygienists in the office, I would designate 1 to be the Hygiene team leader. This will give your hygienists a voice in your management meetings, someone to ensure that hygiene goals are being met, and give you 1 point person to work with in regards to your hygiene systems.

With 3 or more hygienists, you probably already have

someone doing your hygiene coordinating (if you don't you should.) Which allows your hygiene team leader time to work on training and development for the hygiene team.

Once a week, usually on Mondays at Noon, I met with my clinic administrator for 1 hour. The agenda for this meeting is simple.

- What were the highlights of last week?

- Update on where are we in relation to our key performance indicators? These are the numbers we are tracking to ensure we are performing well.

- Update on where are we in relation to our 90-day sprint, which we created by breaking our 1-year strategic goals into quarterly sprints that listed everything that needed to be done.

- Upcoming weeks highlights, anything that I need to be aware of

- What isn't working and what is the plan to fix it – are we tweaking a system, creating a new system, tweaking the current team.

- Discuss the topics for the weekly team meetings

As your practice continues to grow, you will continue to designate additional team leaders who will then report to your clinic administrator who in turn reports to you.

Allowing you to continue to spend your time on high production dentistry while your practice still runs the way that you have determined.

Let's review the role of each of these potential team leaders:

Clinical Team Lead: They lead the hiring/firing of the clinical team, manage the schedules, vacations and sick days for the team. They become the point person to resolve any problems that arise.

Like the Clinic Administrator, they are a noticer, they notice what can be improved on and they work on to improve it.

In addition, they oversee bonuses for the clinical team.

Their job is accountability to the systems. Is the team following the systems? If not, they provide additional coaching to help them do it.

The clinical team lead is not a full-time job, this is done in addition to their other clinical duties.

Once the team on the clinical side of the practice hits 7+ members, now it's time for an additional leader back there. Asking any one person to manage more than 7 people while doing their job is setting them up for failure

Hygiene Team Lead: Once the clinical team hits 7+, then I add a hygiene team lead. The Hygiene team lead does many of the same things as I just describe for the clinical team leader for the Hygiene team.

They lead the hiring/firing of hygienists, assistants and hygiene coordinators. They will manage the schedules, vacations and sick days for the hygiene team, while resolving any issues that arise.

As with the clinical team lead or administrator, they're also 'noticers.' They notice what can be improved and strive to improve it.

They oversee the bonuses for the clinical team and they provide accountability.

As with the clinical team lead, the hygiene team lead can do this in addition to their other duties until the team grows larger than 7. At that point, they will need to spend more time dedicated to the administrative duties than allowed in a part-time capacity.

Administrative Team Lead: At the point that the Clinic Administrator is managing 7+ people (the clinical team lead, the hygiene team lead, and more than 5 administrative persons) I add an administrative team lead.

They will manage the same pieces as the clinical and hygiene team leads; they lead the hiring/firing of the administrative team, manage the schedules, vacations and sick days for the team. And become the point person to resolve any problems that arise.

Like the other administrators, they are also a 'noticer', they notice what can be improved on and they work on to improve it.

Their job is accountability to the systems. Is the team following the systems? If not, they provide additional coaching to help them do that.

As with the clinical and hygiene team lead, the admin team lead can do this in addition to their other duties until the team grows larger than 7.

Now your clinic administrator is really overseeing 3 people, the clinical team leader, the hygiene team leader, and the administrative team leader. They will be meeting with each team lead once a week for at least an hour, following the same agenda that I follow with the Clinic Administrator.

I go into much greater detail on hiring, in *The Insiders Guide to Hiring The BEST Dental Team* ... *Discover how to hire, train, and retain your ideal dental team.* Available at **www.HireTheBestDentalTeam.com**

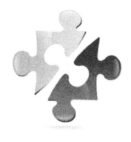

PART 3

GROW WITH PROFITS

CHAPTER 12

Tiger Proof™ Your Practice

By Dr. John Meis

Step #4: "Tiger Proof Your Practice" ™

Once you have maximized your production to extract the added cash that you need (while providing a superior experience and superior care for your patients), and you have created the systems for your practice to grow, and developed your management team, you are ready for Step #4.

You see, everything that we have done up to this point, has made you and your current team more productive. This was the point that I was at when I was producing in the top 1% of the country.

You are reaping the benefits of your increased training,

you and your team have greater skills and if we left it alone at this point, you will have created a monster. Because your practice now relies on you more than ever ... but, at the beginning of this book, I promised you the freedom to be able to enjoy it!

I highly recommend that during your economic boom, the time frame when your production continues to skyrocket, that you are setting aside a portion of that money. Because you are soon going to discover, if you haven't already, that you are running out of capacity.

- Do you have enough treatment rooms?

- Do you have enough people?

- Do you have enough supplies?

- Do you have enough parking spaces?

- Do you have enough computers?

- Do you have enough technology?

- Do you have enough Doctor time?

How do you know when you are running out or have run out of any of the above?

One of the best ways to know, is that the team will tell you, they'll tell you when you need more stuff, they'll tell you when you need more chairs, they'll tell you when you need more hand pieces. They'll tell you when you need more ultra-sonic tips.

When a team member tells you they need something *just get it.* They're telling you that they're out of capacity, that they're waiting around for something or that they don't have enough and it's impeding their production and impeding your revenue. Whatever they tell you they need, just get it.

It's that simple.

Now, how do you know when you are out of Doctor time?

When you are spending only the time that I talked about as a doctor, doing the duties I have talked about and the rest of your time is spent treating patients, with no downtime.

When you can answer the following questions:

• Have you delegated all non-treatment to other team members?

• Are you spending an hour or less with your clinic administrator? (and spending the rest of the time treating patients)

- Are your only non-clinical duties; your daily huddle, your weekly team meeting, overseeing accounting and your checkbook, and strategic planning?

At this point you're out of doctor capacity, you are <u>out of you</u>. Your practice can no longer grow due to the fact that you will be holding them back.

- At the end of your day do you feel mentally fatigued or like you could go for another hour or 2?

- Do you come into work excited about the day?

If you are not feeling engaged, if you are not coming into work every day excited about what the day is about to bring, you have started to struggle with the emotional load.

You have reached the capacity of your mental and emotional abilities and if that doesn't change, your practice (and dentistry) will suffer.

This is a little harder to predict. It could happen to you at $70,000 a month or it might not happen until you reach $200,000 a month. For every doctor it is different, and the important piece is being able to recognize it and put step #4 into place before you go over the edge.

It is at this point, that we can start the process of Tiger Proofing™

Do you remember, not that long ago, when Siegfried and Roy were THE show in Las Vegas? They performed every night to sold out crowds from 1990 until the fateful night October 3, 2003.

At the same time, a group known as "The Blueman Group" also started performing.

What was the difference?

On that fateful October night, Siegfried and Roy discovered what many Dentists discover – that if one of the 2 stars of their show were no longer there, they no longer had a show.

Unfortunately the same holds true for many dental practices. If the dentist were to suffer a medical set-back or wanted to retire, the practice suffers immediately.

If a blueman were to have an experience like Siegfried had, they would simply add in a new man and paint his face blue and the show would go on.

You have built up enough capacity to adequately supply another provider, and the best part, is that you have also built up a highly productive team to support this additional provider ☺

Why would you want to add in an associate?

In addition to the chance that you could be eaten by a tiger, 'tiger proofing' your practice is the BIGGEST step that you can take toward financial freedom. Because as long as the practice relies on you as the largest source of production, you have only built yourself a JOB.

True financial freedom comes when you are able to passively make income

To completely *Tiger Proof* yourself, it will mean that you are replaceable only when you want to be replaced.

You can continue to practice until your hearts content, all while knowing that should you want to stop practicing for any reason, you can do so.

CHAPTER 13

How Do You Hire An Associate?

By Dr. John Meis

Before bringing on an associate, you want to ensure that both you and your practice are ready. Are you both physically and emotionally prepared to have another dentist in your practice?

Here is the checklist that I use to determine if a practice is ready and guide those that are ready to set their associate up for success.

☐ Do you have enough new patient flow to feed an associate?

☐ Are you willing to improve your own marketing skills?

☐ Are you willing to increase your marketing budget?

☐ Do you have a positive track record of bringing in new patients?

☐ Do you have enough capacity to support an associate?

☐ Is your team excelling at providing same-day dentistry treatments?

☐ Do you have a Clinic Administrator managing the practice?

☐ Are you willing to hire additional team members?

☐ Are you willing to take on the responsibility of doing what you need to do to help an associate succeed?

☐ Are you willing to give a greater share of the new patients to the associate?

☐ Are you willing to do what no one did for you?

☐ Are you willing to give your associate your best assistant?

☐ Are you willing to take a dip in your income while your associate ramps up?

There are a few keys to creating a highly effective associate relationship

Key #1: You bring on an associate once your practice is ready. Those that bring on an associate before their practice is properly set up rarely succeed. This is why we always start by maximizing productivity and training both the owner/doctor and the team to be highly proficient in their daily activities. (plus the extra revenue is an added boost to help us in our journey)

Now we have systems in place to be able to present same-day dentistry and have worked our practice until we are approaching a capacity crisis.

At this time, we are ready for an associate. We have set up systems to ensure that we can not only bring in another provider, but we can bring in additional team members and the practice won't miss a beat.

It is at this time, that a new associate will be able to come into the practice, have a place to practice and have patients to treat.

They are not capable of this without you (that's why they are choosing to be an associate) and they are looking for you to mentor them.

If you were to bring in an associate, and you didn't have patients for them to treat or a place for them to treat, you would only be setting each other up for failure.

Key #2: You hire a good fit for your practice: I am always looking for an associate (or any team member) who is looking for an opportunity not security. The questions that you ask during this phase should shed light on their true intentions.

I look at their past experiences – are they moving from one bad experience to the next? If I hire them will I be their next bad experience? Past experiences are a good indicator of future success.

I compare philosophies – it's great to have a conversation about procedures and philosophies, because not everyone has the same philosophy. If you are going to be working with someone, your philosophies and your ideas about procedures need to be in line. The last thing that you want is to confuse patients with 2 different treatment philosophies…. Confused patients run for the door.

I look at their ability to work as a team member – do they see themselves as a team member? You just spent all this time and resources setting your team up for success and creating these systems to have a team run practice. A doctor walking in thinking that they are above everyone else will derail everything you have done to this point.

Are they willing and able to do what ever it takes to get what needs to be done done? After all, if some of these ideas are new to you; hygiene productivity, same-day-dentistry, a team run practice, you can be sure that they will also be new to an associate. Are they willing to try new things or is their way the only way?

Key #3: You set your associate up for success:

Did you catch the question? Are you willing to give your associate your best assistant?

Associate doctors are young and inexperienced. They don't know your treatment philosophies (another reason having a system for your tribal language and case presentation are so important.)

When you hire a new assistant, who is inexperienced, to work with an inexperienced associate in the crappy rooms, that is not setting that person up for success. If you do that … everyone is likely to fail.

As much as it pains me, I give every new associate my best assistant.

Why?

Because that assistant has been trained on our systems, she can lead the associate when I might not be able to. She can help them work our systems to be the most productive and provide the optimal care for their patients.

The associates learning time is cut in half, when they are given every possible head start.

CHAPTER 14

How Do You Replace Your Salary With Profits?

By Dr. John Meis

Before we talk about replacing your salary, let me ask you a question...

How do you currently pay yourself?

Are you paid as a provider in your practice or at the end of the month do you pay all the bills, pay all the salaries, and then anything that is left over is your pay for that month?

When you wait to pay yourself at the end of the month, hoping that there is money left over, you are running your practice as though it is your job.

I know, it's an odd way of thinking about it, after all, if it was a 'job' wouldn't you have a salary? When you start to run your practice as a business you start to think about it differently.

Have you ever heard the financial guru's say that they only way to true wealth is to pay yourself first? It's part of the reason that 401K's were created – to help people pay them selves first.

As a business owner, your potential to pay yourself first is multiplied! You should be taking advantage of every possible way of paying yourself first.

The first thing is to ensure that you are paid as a provider in your practice. If your associate is being paid a salary plus a percentage of collections, you should have that same structure for yourself. Now, everything that is left over at the end of the month is true business profit.

And here is where it becomes fun… as the owner doctor those business profits are a second stream of income. Now as the production grows, your profit will also grow and your business profits will continue to grow. As you add in more providers and their production grows, your business profits grow.

Now, over time, you can produce less, and as long as the practice maintains the production level, you will maintain your income ☺.

CHAPTER 15

Multiple Practices ... Multiple Incomes

By Dr. John Meis

With a good set of systems, and additionally trained providers, you will reach another point of capacity and you have yet another choice. There is no longer room in your practice to add additional providers to bring in additional profit.

You can either:

1. Retire from practicing, and operate as the business owner, freeing up production time for your associate or
2. Expand to multiple practices to continue to add additional providers.

Danger .... Danger .... Danger

This is an advanced strategy – do not try this at home. This is to be done by professionals only. This is how Dentists get into financial trouble. By attempting to expand their practice before they are ready.

** Warning this is an advanced strategy**

Most doctors think that they can just deploy some of their team to a new office and everything will just work. That is the farthest from the truth. Moving people will mean that you have depleted the talent pool in your flagship location, there are no systems set up in your new location and your dentists can't be in 2 places at one time.

If you think that you are ready to expand multiple locations, you should have:

☐ A first location is very profitable. I like to use 15% EBITDA as a benchmark, and your accountant can provide that number for you.

☐ You have documented systems for everything listed in chapter 10

☐ You have a Clinic Administrator PLUS an extra Clinic Administrator already trained and functioning in that role.

☐ You have a Doctor that has been <u>trained on your systems</u> and has been practicing at your current location for a minimum of 6 months that you will be transitioning into your second location.

☐ You are willing to move some of your best team members to your new location.

Advice To Any Dentist Thinking Of Expanding To Multiple Practices

I am often asked what I would say to anyone thinking of expanding to multiple practices and that is:

Create a great team before you go to location #2!

The team includes the obvious people like; your dental office team and your Clinic Administrator . But you are also going to want to have a banker, an attorney, an accountant, a dental supply rep, contractor, realtor, an office designer and decorating team. You will need to have all of those in place because they're going to be doing the legwork for you.

Remember, you've cranked your own productivity so you're busy. By the end of the day, you are spent. You're not going to have a whole lot of time or mental energy to spend on this.

You have to have a great team.

Location #2 is much harder than location #3. I

promise, they get easier every one after this first one. Location #2 is tough, without a great team it's even tougher.

The last piece is choosing the location for the second practice. The old adage of location, location, location, **is the most important decision**.

There are many things that I look for in location but the two that I find most frequently missing from a potential location are:

1. **Plenty of parking:** You should have 3 parking spaces for every dental chair ... that's not easy to find.

2. **The ability for great signage:** That means sign on the exterior of the building, sign with the roadside (either a monument sign or a pole sign.)

If I can't get plenty of parking, and I can't get great signage, I'm not going to do anything in that location.

CHAPTER 16

Why Other Practices Will Struggle And You Won't

Here is where things get really interesting. Most practices don't maximize their hygiene; they don't do same-day-dentistry; they don't create true systems to allow for growth.

They live and die by bringing in new patients...hoping they will wait for an appointment...hoping they will come back in for additional treatment, hoping that they will accept their treatment plans.

Hope is not a strategy – but these 5 keys are.

1. Optimize Production
2. Create Systems for Success
3. Build a Management Team
4. Tiger Proof Your Practice ™
5. Replace Your Salary With Profits

This is why they struggle and you won't.

Let's do the math

The numbers won't lie

- Let's assume your average hygiene production per day is $600 (the current national average) and you have 16 hygiene days a month

- You now increase your hygiene production by 50% (remember, most practices double their production)

- You now produce an increase of $300/day or **$57,600 a year** (and that is for just one hygienist)

- ➤ Let's assume that your current daily Doctor production is $350/hour (the current national average) and you work an average of 128 hours a month

- ➤ You now increase your daily production by 50%* (which is on the low end of possibility, as many see up to 3x as much when implementing the 5-Step Process described here today)

- ➤ You now produce an increase of $175/hour or **$268,800 a year**

When we combine both the hygiene production and doctor production we are now seeing an **increase of $326,400 in production** for the practice.

This is the exact system we apply to every practice that coach or consult with.

We know why you are frustrated. You're frustrated because you don't know WHY you are you are doing what you are doing…. Every day, every marketing strategy, every action isn't a part of a big picture of practice growth.

Every tactic is useless without a system.

I've held nothing back. It's all here for you.

Application of any of these steps in your practice will grow your practice. BUT this process doesn't happen overnight – which is why our coaches work with a practice for a minimum of 12 months usually 24-36 to ensure that the entire 5-step process is up and running in the practice.

Applying this system is what will make you unstoppable

It may seem like a lot right now, but in reality, there are only 5 key steps needed to create the life you have dreamed of. We are speaking from other side.

This is exactly what Dr. John did in his practice, and what I have done in every practice I have gone into.

If, the shy kid from Sioux City Iowa, whose practice was built in the blue-collar capital of the Midwest can do this, I know you can do it.

Think about this for a moment? What if you just did one thing from this book? What would that mean to your practice?

Start today, start with just one thing, BUT START.

Why do we start with increasing your current production?

1. This is area of the practice that can see IMMEDIATE profit and, when done properly, has acceptance rates close to 90%.

2. You can then take this increase in profits and revenue and use it to provide your spring board for Step #2 – so in essence you have invested no additional money into your practice growth and are simply re-investing your profit.

Team Training Institute Certified Coaches and In-Office Training: After going through our Practice Analysis Amplifier, we will create a custom road map to double your practice production.

You will be assigned a personal hygiene coach who will come into your office, train your team and implement your hygiene profit machine. This coach will then work with you and your team monthly to keep your machine rolling. You will also be assigned an Administrative coach who will be responsible for working with you and your team to build your leadership team and the systems required to grow the practice and maintain your growth.

To apply for this level of coaching, call our office at 877-732-2124.

ABOUT THE AUTHORS

Wendy Briggs, RDH has been called the world's most famous Hygienist of all time. She is a practicing hygienist, strategic advisor, speaker, trainer, consultant and coach. She has directly influenced more than 3,718 dental practices in 12 countries around the world. She has the longest track record of doubling hygiene production.

She has consulted and worked with some of the biggest and fastest growing private dental practices, as well as some of the largest DSO organizations in both the United States and Australia, including Heartland Dental, Mortenson Dental & Dental Corp.

As a speaker, she has shared the stage with every "name" in dentistry including; Dr. Tom Orent, Woody Oakes, and The Dawson Academy. She has appeared at Chicago Midwinter, the Yankee Dental Meeting, The Greater New York Dental Meeting, The Townie Meeting, Rocky Mountain Dental Implant Institute, The Big Apple Meeting, CDA in San Francisco, the Laser Clinician's Meeting, the Academy for General Dentistry.

Her own conferences have included Bill Rancic, James Malinchak (The Secret Millionaire), Rulon Gardner (Olympic Gold Medalist), Larry Gelwix, Dr. Justin Moody and Samantha Meis (from Shark Tank).

Hygiene is her passion ... and exploding hygiene productivity, case acceptance, and profits are her areas of expertise.

Dr. John Meis is a 4th generation dentist who's been said to have "dentistry in his blood"... LITERALLY. He is an innovator in practice management, marketing, leadership, and team development. He's spent the better part of the last 8 years as one of the top 1% of producers in the United States. He's multiplied his 1 practice into 6. He is a partner in more than 150 dental practices, playing a key role, visiting, coaching and innovating ON THE GROUND inside these practices.

Dr. John's personal production record is $225,000 in just one month.

He's the father of 2, His daughter Samantha has even appeared on the television show Shark Tank securing a partnership with Mark Cuban. He's also a Fellow in the Academy of General Dentistry (FAGD), Diplomat of the International Congress of Oral Implantologists (DICOI).

The Team Training Institute is based in Salt Lake City, should you wish to contact either Wendy or Dr. John Meis about speaking, consulting or just your comments about the book, you call their office at 877-732-2124 or email support@theteamtraininginstitute.com

The Most Incredible Free Gift Ever….

Claim Your $2,998 Dental Practice Growth Gift

Valid for 1 60-minute Practice Analysis Amplifier. The Team Training Institute will analyze your current practice and provide you with a roadmap to implement all 5 key areas of growth in your practice.

To CLAIM Your Gift:
www.HowToDoubleProduction.com/freegift

Made in the USA
Monee, IL
03 July 2024

60895960R00079